BEST NCLEX NOTES

Therapeutic Communication Strategies Vol.1

THE ART OF MASTERING NCLEX QUESTIONS

BY THE NCLEX MASTER

Best Nclex Notes
Therapeutic Communication Strategies Vol.1
The Art of Mastering Nclex Questions
By The Nclex Master

Copyright© 2013 by Regional Hands Inc./ The Nclex Master
All rights reserved, including the right to reproduce this book or any portions in any form whatsoever, without permission in writing from the author.

Disclaimer: Due to the fact that the field of nursing is constantly changing, it is the reader and purchaser's responsibility for doing the research and studying on their own. Also to obtain current health care information. Positive results are individualized. This book is in no way telling or recommending that it is not necessary to study course material provided by the school of their choosing in order to be a successful student and pass a test. This guide is solely for educational and entertainment purposes. Nor does the writer either or publisher of all volumes of this book assume any liability from any injury, damage, negative test results, directly or indirectly to persons either or properties arising from the publication of this book.

Nor does the author either or publisher have any financial gain from the publishers either or writers of recommended readings that are mentioned below.

My references and recommended reading material to utilize throughout nursing school: Saunders Comprehensive Review for the Nclex-RN examination by Linda Anne Silvestri edition 5. Philadelphia. 2005,WB Saunders.
Saunders Strategies for Success for the Nclex-RN examination

ISBN-13: 978-1494322199
ISBN-10: 1494322196

In loving Memory of Anderson F. Redding and Yvonne Lee.

CONTENTS

Introduction..7

Section 1 The Classroom..9

Section 2 Medical Terminology.......................................11

Section 3 Anatomy and Physiology.................................17

Section 4 Nclex Comprehensive Review.........................21

Section 5 Therapeutic Communication Strategies................28

INTRODUCTION

Never before will you have access to helpful tips on Nclex, Hesi, and Ati questions the way I set forth. No matter what quarter you are attending in nursing school; you may have the same feelings that other students around you are experiencing. You also may be asking yourself,

"How well will I do on a nursing exam?"

"Why am I struggling when I am studying hard?"

"How can I master Nclex questions?"

"Will I pass Hesi and Ati exams?"

"Will I pass my school's exit exam?"

"Will I pass my state board exam on the first try?"

These are all valued questions and feelings to have. You can and will reach your goal of becoming a nurse. You just have to make sure you put the knowledge you gain each and every day to work in your best interest.

Be positive; look in the mirror and say, "I am a nurse!"
I have experience some of the same feelings many of you have and I want you to know these 3 things:

I am You.

I was You.

I Am a Nurse.

This book is only one of many different guides that I will provide to you and other nursing students. In the near future there will be several more just like this, but with different topics and test taking strategies to look forward to.

The key is to master one guide at a time. This will help you to be more successful in answering not only nclex questions, but to know what the key elements you need to pay closer attention to, so you can be directed to the correct option.

Please do not take the information or recommendations I give you lightly. Make sure you study the material your professors give you and try your best to comprehend what you are reading. You may also find that you will have trouble understanding some content because it is hard to visualize something that you are not experienced in. When this happens, you really need to dig into nclex questions from the online material and the nclex books. When answering the questions, make sure you read the rationales to the questions. This is a great study tool and it provides you with follow up information that you may not have remembered or understood from your reading materials.

What you will find in all my guides are things you must know and also very helpful hints on the things you do not know to help you answer the questions. You have enough to read in the program itself, this is why my study guides are short and to the point, I am not here to teach you a nursing class, so please read every page carefully, so you can understand what I am referring to. Good Luck!

Section 1

The Classroom

I have been in a classroom full of students and as time would go on, the class would become smaller and smaller. I would ask myself, "What in the world is going on? Why are so many students failing or dropping out?" I will admit that it was hard at times staying positive, when I myself had many doubts. Over and over I would hear my teachers and also read numerous books that told us to get rest, study smarter not harder, and eat a well balance diet. Easier said than done. Let's face it…most of us are adults going back to school, married, divorced, have children, or have other financial obligations. We do not have the luxury of getting enough rest, time to read every single chapter, answer all the questions in every workbook, do extra questions, in addition to making sure we study the lesson plan, and making sure we hand in homework on time.

You may also encounter some professors who will tell you to study, keep up with your assignments, don't get behind, but all at the same time never tell you what you have to do with the information before you or how to convert it into a passing grade. They don't give you the added information to make your learning more mindful, or should I say what needs to be done to be an effective learner while in nursing school and beyond.

At one point in your class, I want you to look to your left and look to your right, and look all around you. Your class may be full now, but when you get ready to graduate it will probably be cut in half. I am hoping to change this. This is my one of many goals. With our country facing a nursing shortage, I would like to see more students graduate nursing school. You will find out later that the nclex world is a perfect world, and when you actually work in the health field, you will see that the two worlds seem to be totally different than what you were use to in school. The nclex world is like everything else in life. You have to learn the correct way of doing things before you start finding a shorter and quicker route to obtain that same goal. Don't worry about if you have enough knowledge to put your knowledge into actual nursing practice. School is the foundation and you learn how to be a better nurse when you finally start working as a nurse.

These are some of the reasons why I have decided to take what I have seen and experience firsthand. I share these things with you, not to cripple you, but to help you apply the things I tell you, so you can share it with others, and put it into action to help achieve your goal of becoming a nurse.

HINT

Don't over obsess in taking notes. Learn appropriate abbreviations to take notes. Grouping what you learn is one of the helpful keys to succeed. I will tell you more about
grouping as you read on.

Section 2

Medical Terminology

Rule #1: Go back to the basics, which is Medical Terminology.

If you haven't taken this class or it wasn't a requirement, I want you to find a book at the library or local book store, sit there, study, and utilize their nursing books. This will help keep money in your pocket. Nursing school is expensive enough, so why buy every resource that it is out there? Please take advantage of all the **accurate** free material you can get your hands on.

In my opinion, medical terminology will help you get through at least 5% of your cumulative nursing exams. You will encounter numerous questions with words you have never seen before. It's a lot like knowing greek and latin words. If you know prefixes, stem words, and suffixes, you will know not only learn how to correctly spell and pronounce them, but you will know what the words mean. In some instances, medical terminology will help lead you directly to the correct response when the question gives you a disease or disorder you haven't seen before.

HINT
Some Nclex questions you read will give you a lot of unnecessary information that has absolutely nothing to do with picking out the right option.

Example Question:

A 45 year old female is irritated and lives alone. She complains frequently about mild discomfort in her chest. She is about to undergo a **thoracentesis**. The nurse interprets this type of procedure to be which of the following?

Example Options:

1. The patient needs to lie on her stomach and have her friends and family at her bedside to comfort her.
2. The patient needs to lie supine in bed while the nurse performs percussion all over the body to help remove fluid.
3. This is a surgical puncture to remove fluid in the chest region while the patient is sitting up with arms on a pillow over a bedside table.
4. The patient needs to stand up and jump up and down to help fluid move around.

The correct option is #3.

In this scenario, this is the type of question where your medical terminology will help you answer this question correctly. The word *"centesis"* means a surgical puncture to remove fluid.

Information regarding her age and living situation has absolutely nothing to do with what the question is asking you about, which is the procedure; not the patient's psychosocial status.

HINT

Depending on the category the question falls into, usually you will focus on the patient (client) before equipment, but remember this question asked about the procedure.

You can take what you have learned about medical terminology and build on it in your fundamental class of nursing. It is important to know all of your medical terminology if you can. You may feel that this is a challenge to you. I want you to memorize the following ones I list and try adding to the list as time goes on. I will give you the ones that you will see come up over and over on test questions at school.

Medical terms to know:

- Al, ic…..means pertaining to
- Osis…..means abnormal condition
- Ism…..means condition
- Itis…..means inflammation
- Megaly…..means enlargement
- Centesis…..means surgical puncture to remove fluid
- Tomy…..means cutting into
- Ectomy…..means cutting out
- Encephal…..means brain
- Cardi…..means heart
- Thorac…..means chest
- Pneumon, pulmon…..means lung
- Hepat…..means liver
- Col…..means colon

- Cholecyst…..means gallbladder
- Cyst…..means urinary bladder (don't mix this up with "cyte" which means cell)
- Nephr, ren…..means kidney
- Gastyr, lapar…..means stomach
- Peritone…..means the membrane that surrounds the organs in the abdomen, example: peritoneum
- Hyster…..means uterus
- Orch, orchid…..means testicle
- Rhabdomy…..means skeletal muscle
- arthr…..means joint
- oste…..means bone
- oma…..means mass, tumor
- arteri…..means artery
- thromb…..means clotting
- phleb…..means vein
- leuk…..means white
- erythr…..means red
- hyper…..means excessive
- hypo…..means below, under, not enough

Of course there are many more, but these are the ones that are essential to know. These are the ones you will be tested on in the first part of your nursing classes and fundamental hesi.

I can remember when I took the fundamental of nursing class and luckily for me I was able to pass my fundamental hesi exam with a high score. When I finished my hesi exam, I began to think about the test. I could remember the questions I got wrong and the ones I struggled to answer. I was upset at myself because I was one of those students that took my medical terminology class for granted. I received an "A" in the medical terminology class, but honestly I did the work I needed to do to pass the class. I studied the material just to pass the quizzes and test. I didn't study it to retain the information for later on in the program. No one stressed how important this class was. If only I would have made it a habit to at least make it a part of my daily studying I would have been able to answer questions later in the program that would have made a difference in my overall grade.

Some questions on the hesi exams were questions that were worded in a way that I didn't know what the answer could possibly be. Some questions I had read, I would over analyze it and later regret that I had done so. I had the "when I'm at work syndrome", thinking to myself that nurses do this or that at work. Sometimes it was hard to separate the two. At other times my experience working in the health field, helped me to concentrate more on the areas I wasn't familiar with.

I truly believe that almost 5% of the questions on all of my cumulative exams had to do with medical terminology words. I can remember my professor scheming over certain procedures or told us to read certain chapters, but didn't tell us what material we really had to focus on, which left holes all over the place. For those of you who have been in school for a while can understand what I am talking about. The teachers give you so much homework, chapters to read along with power point slides, that you really don't know what is pertinent for you to know come test time. You may also notice that some of the exams you are given does not reflect your professor's lecture. You have to do your own research to find the answers you are looking for. Let's face it; we have some excellent professors and some not so good professors. I will try my best to continue to write guides and post helpful hints online to help you in your journey to nursing.

Your foundation for nursing starts with medical terminology, not the first actual nursing class you sit in. Please pay close attention to this class or incorporate your day to day studying with medical terminology. If I would have taken it more seriously, it would have helped my learning become a smoother transition to the next class.

HINT

Each class builds on one another. You have to try your best to master one area before going on to the next.

Section 3

Anatomy and Physiology

Rule #2: Know your anatomy and physiology. I believe this is almost 10% of all your cumulative nclex questions you will be asked.

The medical terminology that you have read and memorize will help you with your anatomy portion of the test questions.
Anatomy and Physiology is a key component of nursing.
If you know where the organs in your body are located, what the function of each organ is, then you will understand how medication has an effect on your body. You will also know what signs and symptoms to look for.
The physiology portion of the major organs will help you answer difficult pharmacology questions.

HINT
If you know what the normal is, you will have no problem knowing what is wrong, what isn't right, and what abnormal would be.

If you cannot remember anything from your anatomy class, remember where the major organs of your body are located.

I am going to give you a break down of how you should look at certain organs in your body and how you should study for them. You have to learn to group your work to better prepare yourself for your exams.

Example:

A. Medical Terminology:

"Hepat" means liver.

B. Anatomy:

The liver is located in the upper right quadrant

C. Physiology:

The liver produces bile.

The liver empties/releases this bile in the gallbladder.

D. Pharmacology:

The liver is responsible for drug metabolism.

The liver has enzymes (ALT, AST, Phosphatase, and Bilirubin). These levels will be elevated when there are problems going on. (Review normal ranges so when you are given a lab range in the question and it is too high, you will be able to choose the correct option, for example, choosing the option: Notify the doctor and not choosing the incorrect option: Document the findings.)

If there is too much bilirubin in the blood stream it will cause yellowing of the skin which is called jaundice.

Jaundice can be seen in the whites of the eye and oral mucosa in dark skin individuals.

Infants born with jaundice will be put under a bilirubin light to help rid the jaundice.

E. Medical terminology:
"itis" means inflammation

F. Nursing Class:
Hepatitis A- which can be transmitted from contaminated food.

Hepatitis B, C- which can be transmitted from contaminated blood.

Now you will be able to take a topic like liver and expand on it. You can take it a step further and knowing what the relationship to the brain when levels are high, what medications to give, and so on. I am not trying to rewrite books or teach a nursing class; I am just giving you a better way to study. Remember, grouping your work is a more effective learning tool. The examples above are also things you will see on your nursing test and now that you know some of the things you will encounter, you will be able to prepare for an upcoming exam.

HINT

Once you know the medical terminology, take what you learned and apply it to anatomy and physiology, and so forth. This will help you remember everything that is a normal function of an organ of your body.

Ask yourself the following questions:

- What tests are to be used to look for normal functions and abnormal labs? Then find out...
- What does a patient look like when they are having liver problems? If there is a problem...
- What does a nurse need to do?
- What are the common medications to give?
- What are the adverse reactions of the medication?

- What are the types of surgeries performed?
- What position does a patient need to be in after surgery?
- What are the complications that can arise after surgery?
- What type of dressings does a patient have to have?
- What's a normal finding Post Op?

If you can take each organ in your body and answer those questions, then you are that much closer to having the necessary information to answer the question correctly.

Section 4

Nclex Comprehensive Review

Rule #3: Take advantage of the Saunders Nclex Comprehensive Review book, then work your way to the Sauders Test Taking Strategies book. Read these books from the very beginning to the end. Leave the CDs the book provides for you towards the end of nursing school and right before your state boards.

Combine the books I've mentioned above, along with the online resource that is usually located on the front or back of your nursing text books, register the test book for free on the evolve website, and my test taking strategies that I will provide you in the next section, and you should have no problem passing your exams.

If you find yourself missing most of the questions you answer, keep answering the questions anyway. Make sure you are on study mode for the portion of the test you do online so you can have the chance of reading the rationales to the questions. It will enhance your learning experience. You may find that you retain the information better this way than reading all the time. It will make better sense to you.

Please make sure you read the nclex books as soon as you can; especially their test taking strategies and preferably at the start of your program and then periodically to brush up on them. Make it a part of your everyday learning; this will help you to answer many of the test questions being asked.

These strategies are essential to know by heart. Once you know their test taking strategies, you can apply them to test questions. You will find that this is only half of the battle. You will still need to know other ways to answer questions and this is where my strategies come to play. There will come a time where the nclex strategies will not be helpful to answer the questions. You just have to know the information. I know I am repeating things I tell you. That is another clue that it is important information and should be remembered.

I cannot say this is enough; please make sure you pay attention in class, read chapters you will be addressing in class ahead of time, you will be ahead of the game this way, and once your professor ask the class questions in lecture you will not be totally clueless on what the topic is.

HINT

Answer a minimum of 30 Nclex questions daily. This will show you the style of the Nclex World. These questions are nothing like the ones you are use to from other classes. They are far different than answering questions that you are familiar with. By answering at least 30 questions a day when you start nursing school, it will give you a chance to answer over 20,000 questions by the time you graduate. That doesn't even include test questions or case studies you will be doing. The more questions you answer, the better prepared you will be. Don't wait until the last minute to start answering questions. You will find that no matter what source you are getting questions fro to answer, you will be asked the same question just in several different ways.

Example:

You are taking care of a 73 year old male with hepatitis, which of the following signs and symptoms does the nurse notes as an assessment finding? Select all that apply.

Example:

A 73 year old ale with hepatitis is being discharged to go home. Which of the following statements does the client states that require a need for further teaching?

Again, you will be asked the same question just in different ways. If you apply what I told you about how you should group your work to study, then it will also help when you are being asked these types of questions.

Section 5

Therapeutic Communication Strategies

Rule #5: After you have reviewed therapeutic vs. nontherapeutic techniques and what the definition is in your Saunders Nclex book, then you need to use my guide of therapeutic strategies.

My logic behind exams, whether they are Hesi, Ati, your Exit, or Nclex stateboard, is that your cumulative questions will consist of almost 5% of common sense, almost 5% of medical terminology, almost 10% of anatomy and physiology, 15% of all lab values and medical math, 10% of your overall knowledge for nursing school, and 30% of nclex test taking strategies.

What happened to the other 25%?

What will help you to answer those questions?

The answer to the questions is my test taking strategies. I would give myself a higher percentage, but why brag? (smile)

Question:

What are my test taking strategies?

Answer:

I have developed a better way to understand how to approach each question.

I've learned how to take the information the school teaches and what the nclex books tell you about Physiological needs, Safe and Care Environment, Health Promotion and Maintenance, Psychosocial needs,

ABCs, and Maslow's. What I've discovered are certain similarities and certain patterns that all resources have in common and my guide will help lead you to the correct options. No one has time to analyze how "THEY" come up with the questions they provide and how to apply it to a test question while you are in nursing school. I am sure "They" may not have realized such a pattern that correct responses contain in relation to the question being asked and its' category. No matter the source or system I used to answer nclex questions, I was still able to find these similarities. Along with the information from school and nclex books, I believe my test taking strategies will help guide you to the correct option.

How to use Therapeutic Communication Strategies:

1. Learn the things I've told you in the beginning about medical terminology and anatomy.
2. Know normal lab values.
3. Memorize Saunders test taking strategies.
4. Group what you know.
5. Memorize key words and phrases I tell you about, you will see this in the majority of therapeutic questions, and my strategies will help you answer them correctly.

When you think of answering therapeutic nclex questions, always keep your answers client centered.
It is all about the client.
All about how the client feels.
All about what is in the best interest of the client/patient.
All about client's safety.
All about the client psychosocial needs.
It is not about you; not the nurse.

HINT
Correct responses:
- *Asking a patient what they are willing to learn first.*
- *Asking the client about their understanding of procedures; lab results.*

You will be given several different types of nclex questions, which will give you a different scenario of what is going on.

The following questions are ones I want you to remember as therapeutic questions. You will be given a scenario then usually in the last sentence hides the clue to what category the question falls under. At this time we are going to concentrate on questions that will alert you that they are therapeutic.

Every time you see the following questions I want you to say to yourself, "This is a therapeutic question; this falls into the therapeutic category."

A list of therapeutic Questions:
A. (The scenario of the question) then the question will ask one of the following

1. *The most appropriate response to this client is?*
2. *Most appropriate nursing response is?*
3. *What statement by the nurse is most therapeutic?*
4. *The nurse's best reply would be?*

Make sure you keep this page and the next in clear view when you are practicing answering nclex questions until you memorize which category the question goes into and the key words or phrases to answer them correctly. Once you have master this category and key phases I tell you about, I want you to start weaning yourself form this crutch, and try answering the questions on your own. Then get your copy of volume 2 and do the same until you have acquired all volumes and memorize them.

HINT

Whenever you are answering therapeutic questions, eliminate the options with phrases that generalize a situation, whether it is being recognized in the beginning of the sentence or toward the end of the sentence.

Example #1: There are lots of ways….

Example #2: All people….

Example #3: Most people….

Example #4: The doctor knows what is best for you….

Also eliminate sentences that are trying to convince the client they are in good hands.

Eliminate options with the following key words or phrases:

- Why
- Don't worry
- You will do fine
- You will feel
- Everything will be okay
- It really doesn't
- It doesn't mean
- No longer true
- There is no
- I'm sorry
- I agree
- I know
- I am
- I promise to
- Maybe your family can
- That's not
- Try to be
- You need (choose this as the last resort if there is a client safety issue)
- Does not
- Only
- Never
- All
- The doctor knows best
- Eliminate similar options

When selecting the correct options in the Therapeutic category choose the following phrases:

- Tell me….
- Tell me how you feel….
- What would you like….
- Can you describe your….
- You seem….
- You sound concerned….
- Can you tell me what you understand….
- Can you tell me how you feel….
- Asking the patient what they want to learn first
- Any phrases that ask for the client's permission to do something to or for them.
- Any phrases where the patient asks a question and the nurse restates the question.

What I want you to remember:

Look at the question and ask yourself…

Does this question fall into what I like to call the Therapeutic Category?

Locate the therapeutic question from the choices I gave you.

Circle the question.

Read the options.

Eliminate the words that I told you about.

Choose the option with the key words and phrases I told you to look for.

I wish you luck in your future exams while in nursing school. Master this guide before going to one of my other guides. Please do me the honor and post a comment about this book on my website, other social media sites, or online stores' comment section. All feedback is welcome. All my guides are very short but very informative. I am sure it will help you in your journey to become a successful nursing student.

Contact information: nclexmaster@yahoo.com

thenclexmaster@blogspot.com

Follow on twitter @thenclexmaster

www.ingramcontent.com/pod-product-compliance
Lightning Source LLC
Chambersburg PA
CBHW070731180526
45167CB00004B/1710